WALL PILATES FOR SENIORS

A Safe And Effective Exercise Program For Seniors Citizens To Unlock The Power Of Movement, Improve Flexibility, Balance And Strength

Sarah W. Jowers & James D. Coca

Wall Pilates for Seniors

Copyright © 2023 by Sarah W. Jowers & James D. Coca

Table of Contents

INTRODUCTION

Pilates is a form of exercise that focuses on building strength, flexibility, and balance through a series of controlled movements. It is a safe and effective form of exercise that is suitable for people of all ages and fitness levels, including seniors. As we age, it is important to maintain an active and healthy lifestyle to prevent injury and illness, and to improve overall well-being. Pilates is an excellent way to achieve this goal.

This book is a comprehensive guide to Pilates for seniors. This book is designed to help you of all fitness levels and abilities to improve their physical and mental well-being through the practice of Pilates. Whether you are a beginner or have experience with Pilates, this guide will help you to unlock the power of movement, improve flexibility, balance, and strength using the support of a wall.

The core of the book Is a series of progressive Pilates programming that are specifically designed for seniors. These exercises include easy poses, stretches, and exercises that focus on the legs and hips. These exercises are designed to be easy to perform and to improve flexibility, balance, and strength. They are also designed to be safe and effective for you, so they can be performed without the risk of injury.

The book also includes more advanced programs for those who want to take their practice to the next level. It covers exercises that improve upper body strength and flexibility, and also includes exercises that help to increase balance and stability.

We hope that this guide will provide a valuable resource for seniors looking to improve their physical and mental well-being, increase their flexibility, balance, and strength, and enjoy the benefits of Pilates in a safe and effective way. So, get ready to start your Pilates journey and let's unlock the power of movement together.

☐

CHAPTER 1: UNDERSTANDING WALL PILATES FOR SENIORS

What is Wall Pilates?

Wall Pilates is a unique and innovative approach to traditional Pilates exercises that utilizes a wall as a support system. This method is designed to make Pilates exercises more accessible, safe, and effective for seniors, people with limited mobility, or anyone who is looking for an alternative way to practice Pilates.

Wall Pilates is not just about using a wall as a prop. It's about using the wall as a tool to help you achieve better alignment, stability, and balance. The wall provides an added level of support and guidance, allowing you to focus on your movements and achieve optimal results.

This form of Pilates is also ideal for seniors, who may find it difficult to perform traditional Pilates exercises on the mat. The wall provides a stable surface for them to work against, making it easier to maintain proper form and alignment. Moreover, Wall Pilates is also beneficial for seniors as it helps them to improve their balance, flexibility, and strength, which can help prevent falls.

Wall Pilates also offers a wide range of exercises that target different areas of the body, such as the legs, hips, and shoulders. This makes it a versatile and comprehensive exercise program that can meet the needs of a wide range of individuals.

In conclusion, Wall Pilates is a safe, effective, and accessible form of Pilates that utilizes a wall as a support system. It is perfect for seniors, people with limited mobility, or anyone who is looking for an alternative way to practice Pilates. It offers a wide range of exercises that target different areas of the body, making it a comprehensive exercise program that can meet the needs of a wide range of individuals. With Wall Pilates, you can improve your balance, flexibility, and strength, and achieve optimal results.

How Does It Differ From Traditional Pilates?

Wall Pilates differs from traditional Pilates in a number of ways. The primary difference is the use of a wall as a support system. In traditional Pilates, exercises are typically performed on a mat, with little to no external support. In Wall Pilates, the wall serves as a tool to help individuals achieve better alignment, stability, and balance.

Another difference is the level of accessibility. Traditional Pilates can be challenging for some individuals, particularly those with limited mobility or who are recovering from an injury. The wall provides an added level of support and guidance, making it easier for these individuals to perform exercises safely and effectively.

Wall Pilates also offers a wide range of exercises that target different areas of the body, such as the legs, hips, and shoulders, whereas traditional Pilates is more focused on the core. This makes Wall Pilates a more versatile and comprehensive exercise program that can meet the needs of a wide range of individuals.

Wall Pilates differs from traditional Pilates in several ways:

Support: Wall Pilates utilizes a wall as a support system, which provides an added level of stability and guidance. This allows individuals to focus on their movements and achieve optimal results, especially for seniors or those with limited mobility who may find it difficult to perform traditional Pilates exercises on a mat.

Modification: Wall Pilates allows for modifications and variations of traditional Pilates exercises. This means that exercises can be adapted to suit the individual's needs and abilities, making it more accessible for people of all fitness levels.

Focus: Wall Pilates focuses on alignment, stability, and balance, which are especially important for seniors or those with limited mobility. This can help to prevent falls and injuries, and improve overall function.

Variety: Wall Pilates offers a wide range of exercises that target different areas of the body, such as the legs, hips, and shoulders, making it a versatile and comprehensive exercise program.

Safety: Wall Pilates is a safe form of Pilates as it provides added support and guidance, which helps to prevent falls and injuries.

While traditional Pilates is done on a mat, Wall Pilates allows for a different approach, with the wall as a support system. Both traditional Pilates and Wall Pilates focus on improving flexibility, balance, and strength, but Wall Pilates is more accessible and suitable for seniors or individuals with limited mobility.

17

In summary, while traditional Pilates focuses on mat exercises that target the core, Wall Pilates utilizes a wall as a support system and offers a wider range of exercises that target different areas of the body. It's more accessible, safe, and suitable for seniors, people with limited mobility, or anyone who is looking for an alternative way to practice Pilates.

Benefits Of Wall Pilates For Seniors

Wall Pilates offers a variety of benefits for seniors, including:

Improved balance and stability: The wall provides a stable surface for seniors to work against, making it easier to maintain proper form and alignment. This helps to improve balance and stability, reducing the risk of falls.

Increased flexibility and range of motion: Wall Pilates exercises are designed to stretch and loosen tight muscles, improving flexibility and range of motion. This can help seniors to move more freely and comfortably in their daily lives.

Strengthened muscles and bones: Wall Pilates exercises focus on strengthening the core, legs, and upper body, which can help to improve overall muscle tone and bone density.

Enhanced cardiovascular health: Some Wall Pilates exercises are designed to be low-impact, which makes them suitable for seniors who may not be able to participate in high-impact activities. This can help to improve cardiovascular health and increase endurance.

Improved posture and alignment: Wall Pilates exercises focus on proper alignment and posture, which can help to reduce pain and discomfort in the back, neck, and shoulders.

Reduced stress and anxiety: Wall Pilates is a gentle form of exercise that can help seniors to relax, unwind, and de-stress.

Increased self-confidence and self-esteem: Wall Pilates can help seniors to feel stronger, more flexible, and more capable, which can boost self-confidence and self-esteem.

Socialization: Wall Pilates is a group activity and can help seniors to stay socially active and meet new people, which can be beneficial for their mental and emotional well-being. Overall, Wall Pilates is a safe, effective, and accessible form of exercise that offers many benefits for seniors. It can help them to improve their balance, flexibility, strength, cardiovascular health, and overall well-being.

Guiding Principles

There are several guiding principles that are essential for a successful Pilates practice, especially for seniors. These principles are designed to ensure that the exercises are safe, effective, and tailored to the specific needs of the individual.

Proper form and alignment: Pilates exercises are designed to be performed with proper form and alignment to ensure that the exercises are safe and effective. This includes maintaining a neutral spine, engaging the core muscles, and using proper breathing techniques.

Focus on the core: Pilates exercises focus on strengthening the core muscles, which are essential for maintaining balance and stability. This is especially important for seniors, as a strong core can help to reduce the risk of falls and injuries.

Gradual progression: Pilates exercises should be performed in a gradual progression to ensure that the body is prepared for more advanced exercises. This is especially important for seniors, as their bodies may not be able to handle more advanced exercises right away.

Adaptability: Pilates exercises can be modified to suit different levels of fitness and physical limitations. This is especially important for seniors, as they may have chronic conditions or limited mobility.

Mindfulness and breath control: Pilates emphasizes the importance of mindfulness and breath control. This helps seniors to focus on the present moment, reduce stress, and improve overall well-being.

Precision: Precision is an essential aspect of Pilates. The exercises are designed to be performed with precision, which helps to ensure that the exercises are targeting specific muscle groups correctly. Precision also helps to reduce the risk of injury and ensure that the exercises are performed correctly.

Flow: Flow is an essential aspect of Pilates. The exercises are designed to be performed with flow, which helps to promote relaxation and reduce stress. Flow also helps to reduce the risk of injury and ensure that the exercises are performed correctly.

When practicing Pilates, it is essential to focus on these principles to ensure that the exercises are performed correctly and safely. By focusing on proper alignment, breath control, centering, concentration, control, precision, and flow, seniors can ensure that they are getting the most out of their Pilates practice and reaping all the benefits that Pilates has to offer.

In addition to these principles, it is also essential for seniors to listen to their bodies and take the necessary modifications when needed. Pilates is a low-impact form of exercise, but seniors should always be mindful of their body's limitations and make adjustments accordingly.

CHAPTER 2: PREPARING TO EXERCISE

Make A Commitment To Pilates

Making a commitment to Pilates can be a life-changing decision for You. Pilates is a safe and effective form of exercise that can help seniors to improve their flexibility, balance, and strength, while also promoting relaxation and reducing stress. However, making a commitment to Pilates can be difficult, especially for seniors who may have limited mobility or other health concerns.

The first step in making a commitment to Pilates is to understand the benefits of the practice. Pilates is a low-impact form of exercise, which means that it puts less stress on the joints and is less likely to cause injury. This makes Pilates a great form of exercise for seniors who may have limited mobility or other health concerns. Pilates also promotes relaxation, which can help seniors to reduce stress and tension, and can also improve overall well-being.

Once seniors understand the benefits of Pilates, they can then set realistic goals for their practice. Setting goals can help seniors to stay motivated and committed to their Pilates practice. For example, seniors can set a goal to improve their flexibility, balance, or strength, or to reduce stress and tension.

Another important aspect of making a commitment to Pilates is to be consistent with the practice. Consistency is key to achieving results and seniors should aim to practice Pilates on a regular basis. This can be challenging for seniors who may have busy schedules or other commitments, but setting aside even a few minutes a day for Pilates can make a big difference in the long run.

Making a commitment to Pilates also requires patience. Pilates is a form of exercise that requires patience and persistence, and you should not expect to see immediate results. It takes time and dedication to see the benefits of Pilates, but with patience and persistence, seniors will be able to achieve their goals.

Finally, it's important for seniors to remember that Pilates is a lifelong practice, and there is no end to the learning and improvement. Pilates is not only about achieving a certain level of flexibility or strength, but it is also about the journey and the process of learning and improving.

What You Need To Begin

When beginning a Pilates practice, there are a few key items that are necessary to ensure a safe and effective workout. These include:

1. A mat: A Pilates mat is a must-have for any Pilates practice. A mat provides cushioning and support for the body, and it helps to protect the joints. A mat also helps to provide a non-slip surface for the exercises. It is important to choose a mat that is thick enough to provide adequate cushioning, and that is made of a durable, non-slip material.

2. A wall: As the title of the book is Wall Pilates for Seniors, having a wall is essential. A wall provides support and stability for the exercises, which is especially important for seniors. It is important to choose a wall that is sturdy and free of any obstacles that could get in the way of the exercises.

3. Comfortable clothing: It is important to wear comfortable, non-restrictive clothing when practicing Pilates. Clothing that is too tight or restrictive can make it difficult to perform the exercises correctly, and it can also

be uncomfortable. Loose-fitting clothing that allows for a full range of motion is ideal.

4. Water: Staying hydrated is important for any exercise program, and Pilates is no exception. It is important to have water on hand to stay hydrated throughout the workout.

5. A towel: A towel can be helpful for wiping away sweat and keeping the mat clean. It is also helpful to have a towel on hand to use as a prop in certain exercises.

6. A resistance band or small ball: These items can be used to add resistance to certain exercises, which can help to increase muscle strength and tone.

It is also important to consult with a healthcare professional before starting a Pilates practice, especially if you have any medical conditions or concerns. A healthcare professional can help to determine if Pilates is appropriate for you and can provide guidance on modifications for any specific needs.

Additionally, it is important for you to start slowly and gradually increase the intensity and duration of their Pilates practice. Starting with a few basic exercises and gradually building up to more advanced exercises can help to reduce the risk of injury and ensure that the body is ready for the increased demand.

It is also important for seniors to listen to their bodies and take necessary breaks when needed. Pilates should not be painful, and if any exercise causes pain or discomfort, it should be modified or avoided.

Learn The Language

When starting a Pilates practice, it is important to familiarize yourself with the language and terminology used in the exercises. This can help to ensure that you are performing the exercises correctly and getting the most out of your practice. Some key terms to be familiar with include:

1. Core: The core muscles are the muscles that surround the spine and support the body. These muscles include the abdominal muscles, the muscles of the lower back, and the muscles of the hips.

2. Pilates principles: The Pilates principles include proper alignment, breath control, centering, concentration, control, precision, and flow. These principles are the

foundation of the Pilates method, and they are essential for achieving optimal results.

3. Mat work: Mat work is the series of exercises that are performed on a mat. These exercises are designed to target specific muscle groups and improve overall fitness and well-being.

4. Reformer: A reformer is a piece of Pilates equipment that is used to add resistance to exercises. It consists of a sliding carriage that is attached to a series of ropes and pulleys.

5. Contrology: Contrology is the term that Joseph Pilates used to describe his method. It emphasizes the importance of control, proper alignment, and breathing in the exercises.

6. Centering: Centering refers to the process of finding the center of the body and connecting to the core muscles. This is an essential aspect of Pilates, as it helps to ensure proper alignment and stability in the exercises.

7. Breath control: Breath control is an essential aspect of Pilates. The exercises are designed to be performed with

proper breath control, which helps to promote relaxation and reduce stress.

8. Planks: Planks are exercises that involve holding the body in a push-up position, with the hands and toes on the ground. These exercises are designed to strengthen the core and improve stability.

9. Supine: Supine refers to lying on the back.

10. Prone: Prone refers to lying on the stomach.

11. Extension: Extension refers to movements that involve lengthening the spine or limbs.

12. Flexion: Flexion refers to movements that involve shortening the spine or limbs.

By familiarizing yourself with these terms and concepts, you can ensure that you are performing the exercises correctly and getting the most out of your Pilates practice.

Modifications For Pain & Injuries

When starting a Pilates practice, it is important to consider any pain or injuries that may affect your ability to perform the exercises.

Here are some general modifications for pain and injuries that can be applied to many of the exercises in the book:

1. Use a wall for support: Many of the exercises in the book involve using a wall for support. This can help to reduce the demand on the joints and muscles, and can help to reduce pain and discomfort.

2. Use props: Props such as blocks, blankets, and straps can be used to modify exercises and make them more accessible for seniors with pain or injuries.

3. Reduce range of motion: If an exercise causes pain or discomfort, try reducing the range of motion. This can help to reduce the demand on the joints and muscles and can help to reduce pain and discomfort.

4. Avoid exercises that cause pain: If an exercise causes pain or discomfort, it should be avoided. It is important to listen to your body and take necessary breaks when needed.

5. Consult with a healthcare professional: If you have a specific pain or injury, it is important to consult with a healthcare professional before starting a Pilates practice. They can help you to identify exercises that are safe and appropriate for your condition and may be able to provide additional modifications.

In summary, modifications for pain and injuries are provided in this book to make the exercises more accessible for seniors with pain or injuries. These modifications include using a wall for support, using props, reducing range of motion, avoiding exercises that cause pain, and consulting with a healthcare professional. With the right approach and modifications, seniors can safely and effectively improve flexibility, balance and strength through the practice of Wall Pilates.

CHAPTER 3: GETTING STARTED WITH WALL PILATES

Basic Wall Pilates Positions

Wall Plank

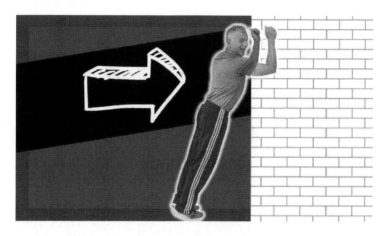

1. Start by facing the wall and placing your hands on the wall at shoulder height, with your palms flat against the wall.

2. Step your feet back until you are in a plank position, with your body forming a straight line from your head to your heels.

3. Engage your core and hold this position for 30-60 seconds.

Benefits: Strengthens the core, shoulders, and upper body.

Wall Push-ups
1. Start by facing the wall and placing your hands on the wall at shoulder height, with your palms flat against the wall.

2. Step your feet back until you are in a plank position, with your body forming a straight line from your head to your heels.
3. Lower your body down towards the wall by bending your elbows, keeping them close to your body.

4. Push back up to the starting position.

5. Repeat for desired number of repetitions.

Benefits: Strengthens the chest, shoulders, and triceps.

Wall Squats

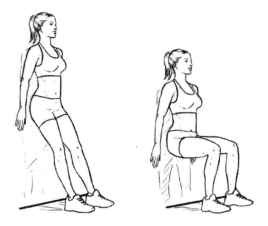

1. Stand facing the wall, with your feet shoulder-width apart.

2. Place your hands on the wall at shoulder height, with your palms flat against the wall.

3. Bend your knees and lower your body down towards the wall as if you were sitting back into a chair.

4. Keep your back straight and your knees behind your toes.

5. Push back up to the starting position.

6. Repeat for desired number of repetitions.

Benefits: Strengthens the legs, glutes, and core.

Wall Lunges
1. Stand facing the wall, with your hands on the wall at shoulder height, with your palms flat against the wall.

2. Step one foot forward and lower your body down towards the wall, keeping your back straight and your front knee behind your toes.

3. Push back up to the starting position and repeat on the other side.

4. Repeat for desired number of repetitions.

Benefits: Strengthens the legs, glutes, and core.

Wall Tricep Dips:

1. Stand facing the wall, with your hands on the wall at shoulder height, with your palms flat against the wall.

2. Step your feet back and lower your body down towards the wall by bending your elbows, keeping them close to your body.

3. Push back up to the starting position.

4. Repeat for desired number of repetitions.

Benefits: Strengthens the triceps and shoulders.

Wall Leg Raises

1. Stand facing the wall, with your hands on the wall at shoulder height, with your palms flat against the wall.

2. Step your feet back and raise one leg up towards the ceiling, keeping the other leg straight.

3. Lower the leg back down and repeat on the other side.

4. Repeat for desired number of repetitions.

Benefits: Strengthens the core and lower abs.

Wall Squat Hold

1. Stand facing the wall, with your feet shoulder-width apart.

2. Place your hands on the wall at shoulder height, with your palms flat against the wall.

3. Bend your knees and lower your body down towards the wall as if you were sitting back into a chair.

4. Keep your back straight and your knees behind your toes.

5. Hold this position for 30-60 seconds.

Benefits: Strengthens the legs, glutes, and core.

Wall Hamstring Curl
1. Stand facing the wall, with your hands on the wall at shoulder height, with your palms flat against the wall.

2. Step your feet back and raise one leg up towards your glutes, keeping the other leg straight.

3. Lower the leg back down and repeat on the other side.

4. Repeat for desired number of repetitions.

Benefits: Strengthens the hamstrings and glutes.

Wall Calf Raises
1. Stand facing the wall, with your hands on the wall at shoulder height, with your palms flat against the wall.

2. Step your feet back and raise up onto your toes, keeping your heels on the ground.

3. Lower your heels back down and repeat.

4. Repeat for desired number of repetitions.

Benefits: Strengthens the calf muscles.

Wall Side Plank

1. Start by facing the wall and placing one hand on the wall at shoulder height, with your palm flat against the wall.

2. Step your feet back and raise your body up onto one hand and the side of your foot, keeping your body in a straight line.

3. Hold this position for 30-60 seconds and repeat on the other side.

Benefits: Strengthens the obliques and core.

Wall Shoulder Taps

1. Start by facing the wall and placing your hands on the wall at shoulder height, with your palms flat against the wall.
2. Step your feet back and raise your body up into a plank position, with your body forming a straight line from your head to your heels.

3. Tap one shoulder with the opposite hand and repeat on the other side.

4. Repeat for desired number of repetitions.

Benefits: Strengthens the shoulders and core.

Wall Chest Fly

1. Stand facing the wall, with your hands on the wall at shoulder height, with your palms flat against the wall.

2. Step your feet back and raise your body up into a plank position, with your body forming a straight line from your head to your heels.

3. Bring your hands together in front of your chest, then open them back up to the starting position.

4. Repeat for desired number of repetitions.

Benefits: Strengthens the chest and shoulders.

Wall L-Sit

1. Sit on the floor with your back against the wall.

2. Place your hands on the floor behind you, with your fingers pointing towards your feet.

3. Raise your legs up so that your body forms an L shape.

4. Hold this position for 30-60 seconds.

Benefits: Strengthens the core and upper body.

Wall Leg Extension

1. Stand facing the wall, with your hands on the wall at shoulder height, with your palms flat against the wall.

2. Step your feet back and raise one leg up towards the ceiling, keeping the other leg straight.

3. Lower the leg back down and repeat on the other side.

4. Repeat for desired number of repetitions.

Benefits: Strengthens the quadriceps.

Wall Leg Press

1. Stand facing the wall, with your hands on the wall at shoulder height, with your palms flat against the wall.

2. Step your feet back and lower your body down towards the wall by bending your knees, keeping them close to your body.

3. Push back up to the starting position.

4. Repeat for desired number of repetitions.

Benefits: Strengthens the legs, glutes, and core.

Wall Abdominal Hold

1. Stand facing the wall, with your hands on the wall at shoulder height, with your palms flat against the wall.

2. Step your feet back and raise your body up into a plank position, with your body forming a straight line from your head to your heels.

3. Engage your core and hold this position for 30-60 seconds.

Benefits: Strengthens the core and improves balance.

Wall Oblique Twist

1. Stand facing the wall, with your hands on the wall at shoulder height, with your palms flat against the wall.

2. Step your feet back and raise your body up into a plank position, with your body forming a straight line from your head to your heels.

3. Twist your body to one side, bringing your elbow towards your hip.

4. Twist back to the starting position and repeat on the other side.

5. Repeat for desired number of repetitions.

Benefits: Strengthens the obliques and improves balance.

Wall Back Extension
1. Stand facing the wall, with your hands on the wall at shoulder height, with your palms flat against the wall.

2. Step your feet back and lower your body down towards the wall by bending your elbows, keeping them close to your body.

3. Push your hips forward and arch your back.

4. Push back up to the starting position.

5. Repeat for desired number of repetitions.

Benefits: Strengthens the back muscles and improves posture.

Wall Back Extension with Arm Raise
1. Stand facing the wall, with your hands on the wall at shoulder height, with your palms flat against the wall.

2. Step your feet back and lower your body down towards the wall by bending your elbows, keeping them close to your body.

3. Push your hips forward and arch your back.

4. Raise your arms up above your head.

5. Push back up to the starting position.

6. Repeat for desired number of repetitions.

Benefits: Strengthens the back muscles, improves posture, and strengthens the shoulders.

Wall Reverse Plank
1. Sit on the floor with your back against the wall.

2. Place your hands on the floor behind you, with your fingers pointing towards your feet.

3. Raise your hips up and straighten your legs, keeping your body in a straight line.

4. Hold this position for 30-60 seconds.

Benefits: Strengthens the core and glutes.

CHAPTER 3: WALL PILATES FOR FLEXIBILITY

Stretching Exercises For The Legs, Hips, And Spine

Wall-assisted hamstring stretch
1. Stand facing a wall, with your feet hip-width apart and about a foot away from the wall.

2. Place your hands on the wall, and step one foot back.

3. Keep your back leg straight and bend your front knee to lower your body towards the wall.

4. Hold the stretch for 20-30 seconds and then switch legs.

The benefits of this stretch include increased flexibility in the hamstrings and lower back, improved posture, and reduced risk of injury.

Wall-assisted hip flexor stretch

1. Begin in a lunge position with your front foot about a foot away from the wall and your back foot behind you.

2. Place your hands on the wall and push your hips forward.

3. Keep your front knee over your ankle and hold the stretch for 20-30 seconds.

4. Switch legs and repeat.

The benefits of this stretch include increased flexibility in the hip flexors and improved posture.

Wall-assisted quad stretch

1. Stand facing a wall, with your feet hip-width apart and about a foot away from the wall.

2. Place your hands on the wall for balance.

3. Bend your knee and bring your heel towards your buttocks.

4. Hold onto your ankle with your hand and hold the stretch for 20-30 seconds.

5. Switch legs and repeat.

The benefits of this stretch include increased flexibility in the quadriceps and improved balance.

Wall-assisted inner thigh stretch

1. Sit on the floor with your legs extended out in front of you.

2. Place the soles of your feet together and bring your heels close to your body.

3. Use your elbows to gently press your knees down towards the floor.

4. Hold the stretch for 20-30 seconds.

The benefits of this stretch include increased flexibility in the inner thighs and improved balance.

Wall-assisted calf stretch

1. Stand facing a wall, with your feet hip-width apart and about a foot away from the wall.

2. Place your hands on the wall for balance.

3. Step one foot back and keep your back leg straight.

4. Bend your front knee and lean into the stretch.

5. Hold the stretch for 20-30 seconds and then switch legs.

The benefits of this stretch include increased flexibility in the calf muscles and improved balance.

Wall-assisted ankle stretch

1. Sit on the floor with your legs extended out in front of you.

2. Place the soles of your feet together and bring your heels close to your body.
3. Use your hands to gently press down on your ankles and hold the stretch for 20-30 seconds.

The benefits of this stretch include increased flexibility in the ankles and improved balance.

Wall-assisted groin stretch

1. Sit on the floor with your legs extended out in front of you.

2. Place the soles of your feet together and bring your heels close to your body.

3. Use your elbows to gently press your knees down towards the floor.

4. Hold the stretch for 20-30 seconds.

The benefits of this stretch include increased flexibility in the inner thighs and improved balance.

Wall-assisted IT band stretch

1. Begin in a lunge position with your front foot about a foot away from the wall and your back foot behind you.

2. Place your hands on the wall and push your hips forward.

3. Keep your front knee over your ankle and hold the stretch for 20-30 seconds.

4. Switch legs and repeat.

The benefits of this stretch include increased flexibility in the IT band and improved posture

Wall-assisted piriformis stretch

1. Sit on the floor with your legs extended out in front of you.

2. Cross one ankle over the opposite knee and sit up tall.

3. Place your hands on the wall for balance and gently press your knee towards the floor.

4. Hold the stretch for 20-30 seconds and then switch legs.

The benefits of this stretch include increased flexibility in the piriformis muscle and reduced risk of sciatic pain.

Wall-assisted glute stretch

1. Sit on the floor with your legs extended out in front of you.

2. Cross one ankle over the opposite knee and sit up tall.

3. Place your hands on the wall for balance and gently press your knee towards the floor.

4. Hold the stretch for 20-30 seconds and then switch legs.

The benefits of this stretch include increased flexibility in the glutes and improved posture.

Wall-assisted low back stretch

1. Begin in a lunge position with your front foot about a foot away from the wall and your back foot behind you.

2. Place your hands on the wall and push your hips forward.

3. Keep your front knee over your ankle and hold the stretch for 20-30 seconds.

4. Switch legs and repeat.

The benefits of this stretch include increased flexibility in the low back and improved posture.

Wall-assisted spinal twist

1. Stand facing a wall, with your feet hip-width apart and about a foot away from the wall.

2. Place your hands on the wall for balance.

3. Turn your torso towards the wall and hold the stretch for 20-30 seconds.
4. Switch sides and repeat.

The benefits of this stretch include increased flexibility in the spine and improved posture.

Wall-assisted spinal extension

1. Stand facing a wall, with your feet hip-width apart and about a foot away from the wall.

2. Place your hands on the wall for balance.

3. Arch your back and hold the stretch for 20-30 seconds.

The benefits of this stretch include increased flexibility in the spine and improved posture.

Wall-assisted spinal flexion

1. Stand facing a wall, with your feet hip-width apart and about a foot away from the wall.

2. Place your hands on the wall for balance.

3. Bend forward and hold the stretch for 20-30 seconds.

The benefits of this stretch include increased flexibility in the spine and improved posture.

Wall-assisted spinal rotation

1. Stand facing a wall, with your feet hip-width apart and about a foot away from the wall.

2. Place your hands on the wall for balance.

3. Turn your torso towards the wall and hold the stretch for 20-30 seconds.

4. Switch sides and repeat.

The benefits of this stretch include increased flexibility in the spine and improved posture.

Wall-assisted neck stretch

1. Stand facing a wall, with your feet hip-width apart and about a foot away from the wall.

2. Place your hands on the wall for balance.

3. Tilt your head towards one shoulder and hold the stretch for 20-30 seconds.

4. Switch sides and repeat.

The benefits of this stretch include increased flexibility in the neck and improved posture.

Wall-assisted shoulder stretch
1. Stand facing a wall, with your feet hip-width apart and about a foot away from the wall.

2. Place your hands on the wall for balance.

3. Reach one arm across your body and hold the stretch for 20-30 seconds.

4. Switch sides and repeat.

Wall-assisted chest stretch
1. Stand facing a wall, with your feet hip-width apart and about a foot away from the wall.

2. Place your hands on the wall for balance.

3. Step one foot back and keep your back leg straight.

4. Bend your front knee and lean into the stretch.

5. Hold the stretch for 20-30 seconds and then switch legs.

The benefits of this stretch include increased flexibility in the chest and improved posture.

Wall-assisted upper back stretch
1. Stand facing a wall, with your feet hip-width apart and about a foot away from the wall.

2. Place your hands on the wall for balance.

3. Step one foot back and keep your back leg straight.

4. Bend your front knee and lean into the stretch.

5. Hold the stretch for 20-30 seconds and then switch legs.

The benefits of this stretch include increased flexibility in the upper back and improved posture.

Wall-assisted full body stretch
1. Stand facing a wall, with your feet hip-width apart and about a foot away from the wall.

2. Place your hands on the wall for balance.

3. Step one foot back and keep your back leg straight.

4. Bend your front knee and lean into the stretch.

5. Hold the stretch for 20-30 seconds and then switch legs.

The benefits of this stretch include increased flexibility in the full body and improved posture.

CHAPTER 4: WALL PILATES FOR BALANCE AND STABILITY

Exercises To Improve Balance And Coordination

Wall-assisted leg swing
1. Stand facing a wall, with your hands resting on the wall at shoulder height.

2. Lift one leg off the ground, and gently swing it back and forth, using the wall for balance.

3. Repeat for 10-15 repetitions, then switch legs.

-Benefits: Improves hip flexibility and strengthens the glutes and hip stabilizer muscles.

Wall-assisted side leg lift
1. Stand facing a wall, with your hands resting on the wall at shoulder height.

2. Lift one leg off the ground, and raise it to the side as high as you can without losing your balance.

3. Repeat for 10-15 repetitions, then switch legs.

-Benefits: Strengthens the hip abductor muscles and improves balance and stability.

Wall-assisted leg press

1. Stand facing a wall, with your hands resting on the wall at shoulder height.

2. Place one foot behind the other, and press your back leg into the wall as you bend the front knee.

3. Repeat for 10-15 repetitions, then switch legs.

-Benefits: Strengthens the quadriceps and improves balance and stability.

Wall-assisted leg extension

1. Stand facing a wall, with your hands resting on the wall at shoulder height.
2. Extend one leg straight out in front of you, and press the heel into the wall.

3. Repeat for 10-15 repetitions, then switch legs.

-Benefits: Strengthens the quadriceps and improves balance and stability.

Wall-assisted leg abduction
1. Stand facing a wall, with your hands resting on the wall at shoulder height.

2. Lift one leg out to the side, and press the outer thigh into the wall.

3. Repeat for10-15 repetitions, then switch legs.

-Benefits: Strengthens the hip abductor muscles and improves balance and stability.

Wall-assisted leg adduction
1. Stand facing a wall, with your hands resting on the wall at shoulder height.

2. Lift one leg and bring it across your body, and press the inner thigh into the wall

3. Repeat for 10-15 repetitions, then switch legs.

-Benefits: Strengthens the hip adductor muscles and improves balance and stability.

Wall-assisted standing leg curl
1. Stand facing a wall, with your hands resting on the wall at shoulder height.

2. Lift one foot off the ground, and bend your knee, bringing your heel towards your buttocks.

3. Repeat for 10-15 repetitions, then switch legs.

-Benefits: Strengthens the hamstrings and improves balance and stability.

Wall-assisted seated leg curl
1. Sit facing a wall, with your hands resting on the wall at shoulder height.

2. Lift one foot off the ground, and bend your knee, bringing your heel towards your buttocks.

3. Repeat for 10-15 repetitions, then switch legs.

-Benefits: Strengthens the hamstrings and improves balance and stability.

Wall-assisted standing leg extension
1. Stand facing a wall, with your hands resting on the wall at shoulder height.

2. Extend one leg straight out behind you, and press the heel into the wall.

3. Repeat for 10-15 repetitions, then switch legs.

-Benefits: Strengthens the glutes and improves balance and stability.

Wall-assisted seated leg extension
1. Sit facing a wall, with your hands resting on the wall at shoulder height.

2. Extend one leg straight out in front of you, and press the heel into the wall.

3. Repeat for 10-15 repetitions, then switch legs.

-Benefits: Strengthens the quadriceps and improves balance and stability.

Wall-assisted standing leg press
1. Stand facing a wall, with your hands resting on the wall at shoulder height.

2. Place one foot behind the other, and press your back leg into the wall as you bend the front knee.

3. Repeat for 10-15 repetitions, then switch legs.

-Benefits: Strengthens the quadriceps and improves balance and stability.

Wall-assisted seated leg press
1. Sit facing a wall, with your hands resting on the wall at shoulder height.
2. Place one foot behind the other, and press your back leg into the wall as you bend the front knee.

3. Repeat for 10-15 repetitions, then switch legs.

-Benefits: Strengthens the quadriceps and improves balance and stability.

Wall-assisted standing leg lift
1. Stand facing a wall, with your hands resting on the wall at shoulder height.

2. Lift one leg off the ground, and raise it as high as you can without losing your balance.

3. Repeat for 10-15 repetitions, then switch legs.

-Benefits: Strengthens the quadriceps and improves balance and stability.

Wall-assisted seated leg lift
1. Sit facing a wall, with your hands resting on the wall at shoulder height.

2. Lift one leg off the ground, and raise it as high as you can without losing your balance.

3. Repeat for 10-15 repetitions, then switch legs.

-Benefits: Strengthens the quadriceps and improves balance and stability.

Wall-assisted standing leg abduction
1. Stand facing a wall, with your hands resting on the wall at shoulder height.

2. Lift one leg out to the side, and press the outer thigh into the wall.

3. Repeat for 10-15 repetitions, then switch legs.

-Benefits: Strengthens the hip abductor muscles and improves balance and stability.

Wall-assisted seated leg abduction
1. Sit facing a wall, with your hands resting on the wall at shoulder height.

2. Lift one leg out to the side, and press the outer thigh into the wall.

3. Repeat for 10-15 repetitions, then switch legs.

-Benefits: Strengthens the hip abductor muscles and improves balance and stability.

Wall-assisted standing leg adduction
1. Stand facing a wall, with your hands resting on the wall at shoulder height.

2. Lift one leg and bring it across your body, and press the inner thigh into the wall.

3. Repeat for 10-15 repetitions, then switch legs.

-Benefits: Strengthens the hip adductor muscles and improves balance and stability.

Wall-assisted seated leg adduction
1. Sit facing a wall, with your hands resting on the wall at shoulder height.

2. Lift one leg and bring it across your body, and press the inner thigh into the wall.

3. Repeat for 10-15 repetitions, then switch legs.

-Benefits: Strengthens the hip adductor muscles and improves balance and stability.

Wall-assisted ankle rotation
1. Stand facing a wall, with your hands resting on the wall at shoulder height.

2. Lift one foot off the ground, and rotate your ankle in a circular motion.

3. Repeat for 10-15 repetitions, then switch legs.

-Benefits: Improves ankle flexibility and strengthens the ankle stabilizer muscles.

Wall-assisted balance walk
1. Stand facing a wall, with your hands resting on the wall at shoulder height.

2. Take small steps forward, using the wall for balance.

3. Repeat for 10-15 steps, then switch direction.

-Benefits: Improves balance and stability, and strengthens the lower body muscles.

Standing And Seated Wall Pilates Exercises

Wall-assisted standing hamstring stretch

1. Begin by standing facing a wall, with your feet about hip-distance apart and your hands resting on the wall for support.

2. Shift your weight to your left foot and raise your right foot behind you, placing the heel on the wall.

3. Slowly bend your left knee, keeping your right leg straight and your heel pressed against the wall.

4. Hold the stretch for 15-20 seconds and then switch sides.

5. Repeat the exercise 2-3 times on each side.

Benefits: This exercise helps to stretch the hamstring muscles, which can become tight and stiff with age. It also improves flexibility and range of motion in the legs, and can help to prevent falls by improving balance and stability.

Wall-assisted standing hip flexor stretch

1. Begin by standing facing a wall, with your feet about hip-distance apart and your hands resting on the wall for support.

2. Place your right foot behind you, with the heel on the wall.

3. Slowly bring your left knee forward, keeping your right leg straight and your heel pressed against the wall.

4. Hold the stretch for 15-20 seconds and then switch sides.

5. Repeat the exercise 2-3 times on each side.

Benefits: This exercise helps to stretch the hip flexor muscles, which can become tight and stiff with age. It also improves flexibility and range of motion in the hips and legs, and can help to prevent falls by improving balance and stability.

Wall-assisted standing quad stretch

1. Begin by standing facing a wall, with your feet about hip-distance apart and your hands resting on the wall for support.

2. Bend your right knee and bring your heel towards your buttocks, grasping your ankle with your right hand.

3. Keep your left leg straight and press your hips forward.

4. Hold the stretch for 15-20 seconds and then switch sides.

5. Repeat the exercise 2-3 times on each side.

Benefits: This exercise helps to stretch the quadriceps muscles, which can become tight and stiff with age. It also improves flexibility and range of motion in the legs, and can help to prevent falls by improving balance and stability.

Wall-assisted standing inner thigh stretch

1. Begin by standing facing a wall, with your feet about hip-distance apart and your hands resting on the wall for support.

2. Step your right foot out to the side, with the heel on the wall.

3. Slowly bend your left knee, keeping your right leg straight and your heel pressed against the wall.

4. Hold the stretch for 15-20 seconds and then switch sides.

5. Repeat the exercise 2-3 times on each side.

Benefits: This exercise helps to stretch the inner thigh muscles, which can become tight and stiff with age. It also improves flexibility and range of motion in the legs, and can help to prevent falls by improving balance and stability.

Wall-assisted standing calf stretch

1. Begin by standing facing a wall, with your feet about hip-distance apart and your hands resting on the wall for support.

2. Step forward with your right foot, keeping your heel on the ground and your toes on the wall.

3. Slowly bend your left knee, keeping your right leg straight and your heel pressed against the wall.

4. Hold the stretch for 15-20 seconds and then switch sides.

5. Repeat the exercise 2-3 times on each side.

Benefits: This exercise helps to stretch the calf muscles, which can become tight and stiff with age. It also improves flexibility and range of motion in the legs, and can help to prevent falls by improving balance and stability.

Wall-assisted standing ankle stretch

1. Begin by standing facing a wall, with your feet about hip-distance apart and your hands resting on the wall for support.

2. Step forward with your right foot and place the ball of your foot on the wall, keeping your heel on the ground.

3. Slowly bend your left knee, keeping your right leg straight and your foot pressed against the wall.

4. Hold the stretch for 15-20 seconds and then switch sides.

5. Repeat the exercise 2-3 times on each side.

Benefits: This exercise helps to stretch the ankle muscles, which can become tight and stiff with age. It also improves flexibility and range of motion in the legs, and can help to prevent falls by improving balance and stability.

Wall-assisted seated spinal twist

1. Begin by sitting with your back against a wall, with your feet flat on the ground and your knees bent.

2. Place your right hand on the wall behind you for support.

3. Slowly twist your torso to the left, keeping your back pressed against the wall and your left hand on your left knee.

4. Hold the stretch for 15-20 seconds and then switch sides.

5. Repeat the exercise 2-3 times on each side.

Benefits: This exercise helps to stretch and release tension in the spine, improving flexibility and range of motion. It also helps to improve circulation and can relieve lower back pain.

Wall-assisted seated spinal extension

1. Begin by sitting with your back against a wall, with your feet flat on the ground and your knees bent.

2. Slowly press your lower back against the wall, lifting your chest and head.

3. Hold the stretch for 15-20 seconds and then release.

4. Repeat the exercise 2-3 times.

Benefits: This exercise helps to stretch and release tension in the spine, improving flexibility and range of motion. It also helps to strengthen the muscles of the lower back and can relieve lower back pain.

Wall-assisted seated spinal flexion

1. Begin by sitting with your back against a wall, with your feet flat on the ground and your knees bent.

2. Slowly press your lower back against the wall, lowering your chest and head towards your knees.

3. Hold the stretch for 15-20 seconds and then release.

4. Repeat the exercise 2-3 times.

Benefits: This exercise helps to stretch and release tension in the spine, improving flexibility and range of motion. It also helps to strengthen the muscles of the lower back and can relieve lower back pain.

Wall-assisted seated spinal rotation

1. Begin by sitting with your back against a wall, with your feet flat on the ground and your knees bent.

2. Place your right hand on the wall behind you for support.

3. Slowly twist your torso to the left, keeping your back pressed against the wall and your left hand on your left knee.

4. Hold the stretch for 15-20 seconds and then switch sides.

5. Repeat the exercise 2-3 times on each side.

Benefits: This exercise helps to stretch and release tension in the spine, improving flexibility and range of motion. It also helps to improve circulation and can relieve lower back pain.

Wall-assisted seated neck stretch

1. Begin by sitting with your back against a wall, with your feet flat on the ground and your knees bent.

2. Slowly tilt your head to the right, bringing your right ear towards your right shoulder.

3. Hold the stretch for 15-20 seconds and then switch sides.

4. Repeat the exercise 2-3 times on each side.

Benefits: This exercise helps to stretch and release tension in the neck muscles, improving flexibility and range of motion. It also helps to relieve neck pain and stiffness, and can improve posture.

Wall-assisted seated shoulder stretch
1. Begin by sitting with your back against a wall, with your feet flat on the ground and your knees bent.

2. Bring your right arm across your chest and press it against the wall.

3. Hold the stretch for 15-20 seconds and then switch sides.

4. Repeat the exercise 2-3 times on each side.

Benefits: This exercise helps to stretch and release tension in the shoulder muscles, improving flexibility and range of motion. It also helps to relieve shoulder pain and stiffness, and can improve posture.

Wall-assisted seated chest stretch
1. Begin by sitting with your back against a wall, with your feet flat on the ground and your knees bent.
2. Bring your right arm across your chest and press it against the wall.

3. Hold the stretch for 15-20 seconds and then switch sides.

4. Repeat the exercise 2-3 times on each side.

Benefits: This exercise helps to stretch and release tension in the chest muscles, improving flexibility and range of motion. It also helps to relieve chest pain and stiffness, and can improve posture.

Wall-assisted seated upper back stretch
1. Begin by sitting with your back against a wall, with your feet flat on the ground and your knees bent.

2. Place your hands behind your head and press your elbows against the wall.

3. Hold the stretch for 15-20 seconds and then release.

4. Repeat the exercise 2-3 times.

Benefits: This exercise helps to stretch and release tension in the upper back muscles, improving flexibility and range of motion. It also helps to relieve upper back pain and stiffness, and can improve posture.

Wall-assisted standing leg press
1. Begin by standing facing a wall, with your feet about hip-distance apart and your hands resting on the wall for support.

2. Place your right foot behind you, with the heel on the wall.

3. Slowly press your right leg against the wall, using your quadriceps muscles.

4. Hold the press for 15-20 seconds and then switch sides.

5. Repeat the exercise 2-3 times on each side.

Benefits: This exercise helps to strengthen the quadriceps muscles, improving muscle tone and endurance. It also helps to improve balance and stability, and can help to prevent falls.

Wall-assisted standing leg extension
1. Begin by standing facing a wall, with your feet about hip-distance apart and your hands resting on the wall for support.

2. Place your right foot behind you, with the heel on the wall.

3. Slowly press your right leg against the wall, using your quadriceps muscles.

4. Hold the press for 15-20 seconds and then switch sides.

5. Repeat the exercise 2-3 times on each side.

Benefits: This exercise helps to strengthen the quadriceps muscles, improving muscle tone and endurance. It also helps to improve balance and stability, and can help to prevent falls.

Wall-assisted standing leg abduction
1. Begin by standing facing a wall, with your feet about hip-distance apart and your hands resting on the wall for support.

2. Step your right foot out to the side, with the heel on the wall.

3. Slowly press your right leg against the wall, using your inner thigh muscles.

4. Hold the press for 15-20 seconds and then switch sides.

5. Repeat the exercise 2-3 times on each side.

Benefits: This exercise helps to strengthen the inner thigh muscles, improving muscle tone and endurance. It also helps to improve balance and stability, and can help to prevent falls.

Wall-assisted standing leg adduction

1. Begin by standing facing a wall, with your feet about hip-distance apart and your hands resting on the wall for support.
2. Step your right foot towards the center, with the heel on the wall.

3. Slowly press your right leg against the wall, using your outer thigh muscles.

4. Hold the press for 15-20 seconds and then switch sides.

5. Repeat the exercise 2-3 times on each side.

Benefits: This exercise helps to strengthen the outer thigh muscles, improving muscle tone and endurance. It also helps to improve balance and stability, and can help to prevent falls.

Wall-assisted seated leg press

1. Begin by sitting with your back against a wall, with your feet flat on the ground and your knees bent.

2. Place your right foot behind you, with the heel on the wall.

3. Slowly press your right leg against the wall, using your quadriceps muscles.

4. Hold the press for 15-20 seconds and then switch sides.

5. Repeat the exercise 2-3 times on each side.

Benefits: This exercise helps to strengthen the quadriceps muscles, improving muscle tone and endurance. It also helps to improve balance and stability, and can help to prevent falls.

Wall-assisted seated leg extension

1. Begin by sitting with your back against a wall, with your feet flat on the ground and your knees bent.

2. Place your right foot behind you, with the heel on the wall.

3. Slowly press your right leg against the wall, using your quadriceps muscles.

4. Hold the press for 15-20 seconds and then switch sides.

5. Repeat the exercise 2-3 times on each side.

Benefits: This exercise helps to strengthen the quadriceps muscles, improving muscle tone and endurance. It also helps to improve balance and stability, and can help to prevent falls. This exercise is also great for those who have difficulty standing for long periods of time, as it can be done seated.

CHAPTER 5: WALL PILATES FOR STRENGTH

Building Muscle Strength And Endurance

Wall-assisted push-ups
1. Stand facing a wall, about an arm's length away from it.

2. Place your hands on the wall at chest level, slightly wider than shoulder-width apart.

3. Lean forward and walk your feet back, keeping your body in a straight line from your head to your heels.

4. Lower your body towards the wall by bending your elbows, keeping your body in a straight line.

5. Push back up to the starting position.

6. Repeat for the desired number of repetitions.

Benefits: This exercise targets the chest, triceps, shoulders, and core. It helps to increase upper body strength, improve posture, and build muscle endurance.

Wall-assisted squats

1. Stand facing a wall, about an arm's length away from it.

2. Place your hands on the wall at chest level.

3. Slowly lower your body towards the wall by bending your knees, keeping your back straight and your weight in your heels.

4. Push back up to the starting position.

5. Repeat for the desired number of repetitions.

Benefits: This exercise targets the quadriceps, hamstrings, glutes, and core. It helps to increase lower body strength, improve balance, and build muscle endurance.

Wall-assisted lunges

1. Stand facing a wall, about an arm's length away from it.

2. Place your hands on the wall at chest level.

3. Step forward with one foot and lower your body towards the wall by bending both knees.

4. Push back up to the starting position and repeat on the other side.

5. Repeat for the desired number of repetitions.

Benefits: This exercise targets the quadriceps, hamstrings, glutes, and core. It helps to increase lower body strength, improve balance, and build muscle endurance.

Wall-assisted tricep dips

1. Stand facing a wall, about an arm's length away from it.

2. Place your hands on the wall behind you at shoulder-width apart.

3. Bend your elbows and lower your body towards the wall.

4. Push back up to the starting position.

5. Repeat for the desired number of repetitions.

Benefits: This exercise targets the triceps, shoulders, and core. It helps to increase upper body strength, improve posture, and build muscle endurance.

Wall-assisted leg raises
1. Stand facing a wall, about an arm's length away from it.

2. Place your hands on the wall at chest level.
3. Slowly lift one leg out to the side, keeping your body in a straight line.

4. Lower back to the starting position and repeat on the other side.

5. Repeat for the desired number of repetitions.

Benefits: This exercise targets the glutes, hamstrings, and core. It helps to increase lower body strength, improve balance, and build muscle endurance.

Wall-assisted squat holds

1. Stand facing a wall, about an arm's length away from it.

2. Place your hands on the wall at chest level.

3. Slowly lower your body towards the wall by bending your knees, keeping your back straight and your weight in your heels.

4. Hold the squat position for the desired amount of time.

5. Push back up to the starting position.

Benefits: This exercise targets the quadriceps, hamstrings, glutes, and core. It helps to increase lower body strength, improve balance, and build muscle endurance.

Wall-assisted hamstring curls

1. Stand facing a wall, about an arm's length away from it.

2. Place your hands on the wall at chest level.

3. Position your heels on top of a small towel or mat.

4. Slowly lift your hips towards the wall by contracting your hamstrings.

5. Lower your hips back to the starting position.

6. Repeat for the desired number of repetitions.

Benefits: This exercise targets the hamstrings, glutes, and core. It helps to increase lower body strength, improve balance, and build muscle endurance.

Wall-assisted calf raises

1. Stand facing a wall, about an arm's length away from it.

2. Place your hands on the wall at chest level.

3. Slowly lift your heels off the ground, contracting your calf muscles.

4. Lower your heels back to the starting position.

5. Repeat for the desired number of repetitions.

Benefits: This exercise targets the calf muscles and helps to increase lower body strength and build muscle endurance.

Wall-assisted side planks
1. Start in a plank position with your hands on the wall, shoulder-width apart.

2. Rotate your body to the side, stacking your feet on top of each other and lifting your top arm towards the ceiling.

3. Hold this position for the desired amount of time.

4. Rotate back to the starting position and repeat on the other side.

Benefits: This exercise targets the core, shoulders, and obliques. It helps to increase core strength, improve balance, and build muscle endurance.

Wall-assisted shoulder taps
1. Start in a plank position with your hands on the wall, shoulder-width apart.

2. Tap one hand to the opposite shoulder, keeping your hips level.
3. Return to the starting position and repeat on the other side.

4. Repeat for the desired number of repetitions.

Benefits: This exercise targets the core, shoulders, and triceps. It helps to increase upper body strength, improve balance, and build muscle endurance.

Wall-assisted chest flys
1. Stand facing a wall, about an arm's length away from it.

2. Place your hands on the wall at chest level, slightly wider than shoulder-width apart.

3. Slowly move your hands out to the sides, keeping your elbows slightly bent.

4. Bring your hands back to the starting position.

5. Repeat for the desired number of repetitions.

Benefits: This exercise targets the chest, shoulders, and triceps. It helps to increase upper body strength, improve posture, and build muscle endurance.

Wall-assisted L-Sit

1. Start in a seated position with your back against the wall.

2. Place your hands on the wall beside you for support.

3. Slowly lift your legs off the ground, keeping your knees bent and your body in an L shape.

4. Hold this position for the desired amount of time.

5. Lower your legs back to the starting position.

Benefits: This exercise targets the core, quadriceps, and hamstrings. It helps to increase core strength, improve balance, and build muscle endurance.

Wall-assisted leg extensions
1. Stand facing a wall, about an arm's length away from it.

2. Place your hands on the wall at chest level.

3. Slowly lift one leg out straight in front of you, keeping your body in a straight line.

4. Lower your leg back to the starting position and repeat on the other side.

5. Repeat for the desired number of repetitions.

Benefits: This exercise targets the quadriceps, hamstrings, and core. It helps to increase lower body strength, improve balance, and build muscle endurance.

Wall-assisted leg press
1. Stand facing a wall, about an arm's length away from it.

2. Place your hands on the wall at chest level.
3. Slowly press one leg out straight in front of you, keeping your body in a straight line.

4. Lower your leg back to the starting position and repeat on the other side.

5. Repeat for the desired number of repetitions.

Benefits: This exercise targets the quadriceps, hamstrings, and core. It helps to increase lower body strength, improve balance, and build muscle endurance.

Wall-assisted abdominal holds
1. Start in a seated position with your back against the wall.

2. Place your hands on the wall beside you for support.

3. Slowly lift your legs off the ground, keeping your knees bent and your body in a straight line.

4. Hold this position for the desired amount of time.

5. Lower your legs back to the starting position.

Benefits: This exercise targets the core, quadriceps, and hamstrings. It helps to increase core strength, improve balance, and build muscle endurance.

Wall-assisted oblique twists

1. Start in a seated position with your back against the wall.

2. Place your hands on the wall beside you for support.

3. Slowly twist your torso to one side, keeping your legs in a straight line.

4. Hold this position for the desired amount of time.

5. Slowly twist back to the starting position and repeat on the other side.

Benefits: This exercise targets the core, obliques, and hip flexors. It helps to increase core strength, improve balance, and build muscle endurance.

Wall-assisted back extensions
1. Start in a prone position with your hands on the wall beside you for support.

2. Slowly lift your upper body off the ground, keeping your legs in a straight line.

3. Hold this position for the desired amount of time.

4. Lower your upper body back to the starting position.

Benefits: This exercise targets the lower back, glutes, and core. It helps to increase lower body strength, improve balance, and build muscle endurance.

Wall-assisted back extensions with arm raise
1. Start in a prone position with your hands on the wall beside you for support.
2. Slowly lift your upper body and one arm off the ground, keeping your legs in a straight line.

3. Hold this position for the desired amount of time.

4. Lower your upper body and arm back to the starting position and repeat on the other side.

Benefits: This exercise targets the lower back, glutes, core, and shoulders. It helps to increase lower body strength, improve balance, and build muscle endurance.

Wall-assisted reverse planks
1. Start in a seated position with your back against the wall.

2. Place your hands on the wall beside you for support.

3. Slowly lift your hips off the ground, keeping your legs in a straight line.
4. Hold this position for the desired amount of time.

5. Lower your hips back to the starting position.

Benefits: This exercise targets the glutes, hamstrings, and core. It helps to increase lower body strength, improve balance, and build muscle endurance.

Wall-assisted plank holds
1. Start in a plank position with your hands on the wall, shoulder-width apart.

2. Hold this position for the desired amount of time.

Benefits: This exercise targets the core, shoulders, and triceps. It helps to increase core strength, improve balance, and build muscle endurance.

Upper Body And Core Exercises

Wall-assisted Pull-ups

1. Stand facing a wall and place your hands on the wall at shoulder height, fingers pointing forward.

2. Step back from the wall until your arms are fully extended and your body is in a plank position.

3. Slowly bend your elbows, bringing your chest towards the wall.

4. Push back to the starting position, fully extending your arms.

5. Repeat for desired number of repetitions.

Benefits: This exercise targets the upper back, shoulders, biceps, and triceps, building muscle strength and endurance in the upper body.

Wall-assisted Rows

1. Stand facing a wall and place your hands on the wall at shoulder height, fingers pointing forward.

2. Step back from the wall until your arms are fully extended and your body is in a plank position.

3. Pull your elbows back towards your sides, squeezing your shoulder blades together.

4. Release and repeat for desired number of repetitions.

Benefits: This exercise targets the upper back and shoulders, building muscle strength and endurance in these areas.

Wall-assisted Shoulder Press

1. Stand facing a wall and place your hands on the wall at shoulder height, fingers pointing forward.

2. Step back from the wall until your arms are fully extended and your body is in a plank position.

3. Push your hands up towards the ceiling, fully extending your arms.

4. Slowly lower back to the starting position and repeat for desired number of repetitions.

Benefits: This exercise targets the shoulders, triceps, and chest, building muscle strength and endurance in these areas.

Wall-assisted Bicep Curls

1. Stand facing a wall and place your hands on the wall at shoulder height, fingers pointing forward.

2. Step back from the wall until your arms are fully extended and your body is in a plank position.

3. Bend your elbows, bringing your hands towards your shoulders.
4. Slowly release and repeat for desired number of repetitions.

Benefits: This exercise targets the biceps, building muscle strength and endurance in this area.

Wall-assisted Tricep Dips

1. Stand facing a wall and place your hands on the wall at shoulder height, fingers pointing forward.

2. Step back from the wall until your arms are fully extended and your body is in a plank position.

3. Slowly bend your elbows, lowering your body towards the wall.

4. Push back to the starting position, fully extending your arms.

5. Repeat for desired number of repetitions.

Benefits: This exercise targets the triceps, building muscle strength and endurance in this area.

Wall-assisted Chest Fly

1. Stand facing a wall and place your hands on the wall at shoulder height, fingers pointing forward.

2. Step back from the wall until your arms are fully extended and your body is in a plank position.

3. Bring your hands together in front of your chest, squeezing your chest muscles.

4. Release and repeat for desired number of repetitions.

Benefits: This exercise targets the chest muscles, building muscle strength and endurance in this area.

Wall-assisted Chest Press

1. Stand facing a wall and place your hands on the wall at shoulder height, fingers pointing forward.

2. Step back from the wall until your arms are fully extended and your body is in a plank position.

3. Push your hands forward, fully extending your arms.

4. Slowly release and repeat for desired number of repetitions.

Benefits: This exercise targets the chest muscles, building muscle strength and endurance in this area.

Wall-assisted Lateral Raises

1. Stand facing a wall and place your hands on the wall at shoulder height, fingers pointing forward.

2. Step back from the wall until your arms are fully extended and your body is in a plank position.

3. Raise your arms out to the sides, keeping them straight and parallel to the floor.

4. Slowly lower back to the starting position and repeat for desired number of repetitions.

Benefits: This exercise targets the shoulders, building muscle strength and endurance in this area.

Wall-assisted Upright Rows

1. Stand facing a wall and place your hands on the wall at shoulder height, fingers pointing forward.

2. Step back from the wall until your arms are fully extended and your body is in a plank position.

3. Pull your hands up towards your chin, keeping your elbows close to your body.

4. Slowly release and repeat for desired number of repetitions.

Benefits: This exercise targets the shoulders and upper back, building muscle strength and endurance in these areas.

Wall-assisted Lat Pull-downs

1. Stand facing a wall and place your hands on the wall at shoulder height, fingers pointing forward.

2. Step back from the wall until your arms are fully extended and your body is in a plank position.

3. Pull your elbows down towards your sides, squeezing your shoulder blades together.

4. Release and repeat for desired number of repetitions.

Benefits: This exercise targets the upper back and shoulders, building muscle strength and endurance in these areas.

Wall-assisted Seated Row

1. Stand facing a wall and place your hands on the wall at shoulder height, fingers pointing forward.

2. Step back from the wall until your arms are fully extended and your body is in a plank position.

3. Pull your elbows back towards your sides, squeezing your shoulder blades together.

4. Release and repeat for desired number of repetitions.

Benefits: This exercise targets the upper back and shoulders, building muscle strength and endurance in these areas.

Wall-assisted Reverse Fly

1. Stand facing a wall and place your hands on the wall at shoulder height, fingers pointing forward.

2. Step back from the wall until your arms are fully extended and your body is in a plank position.

3. Bring your hands together behind your back, squeezing your shoulder blades together.
4. Release and repeat for desired number of repetitions.

Benefits: This exercise targets the upper back and shoulders, building muscle strength and endurance in these areas.

Wall-assisted Plank hold

1. Stand facing a wall and place your hands on the wall at shoulder height, fingers pointing forward.

2. Step back from the wall until your arms are fully extended and your body is in a plank position.

3. Hold this position for desired time

Benefits: This exercise targets the core, shoulders, and upper back, building muscle strength and endurance in these areas.

Wall-assisted Side Plank

1. Stand facing a wall and place one hand on the wall at shoulder height, fingers pointing forward.

2. Step back from the wall until your arm is fully extended and your body is in a side plank position.

3. Hold this position for desired time

Benefits: This exercise targets the core, shoulders, and upper back, building muscle strength and endurance in these areas.

Wall-assisted Russian Twist

1. Sit facing a wall with your back against it, your legs bent, and your feet flat on the floor.

2. Place your hands on the wall at shoulder height, fingers pointing forward.

3. Twist your torso to the left, bringing your right elbow towards the wall.

4. Return to center and repeat on the opposite side.

Benefits: This exercise targets the obliques and core, building muscle strength and endurance in these areas.

Wall-assisted Crunch

1. Sit facing a wall with your back against it, your legs bent, and your feet flat on the floor.

2. Place your hands on the wall at shoulder height, fingers pointing forward.

3. Slowly curl your torso forward, bringing your chest towards your knees.

4. Release and repeat for desired number of repetitions.

Benefits: This exercise targets the abs, building muscle strength and endurance in this area.

Wall-assisted Leg Raise

1. Lie on your back facing a wall, with your legs extended and your hands on the wall at shoulder height, fingers pointing forward.
2. Slowly raise your legs up towards the wall, keeping them straight.

3. Release and repeat for desired number of repetitions.

Benefits: This exercise targets the lower abs and hips, building muscle strength and endurance in these areas.

Wall-assisted Bicycle Crunch
1. Lie on your back facing a wall, with your hands on the wall at shoulder height, fingers pointing forward.

2. Bring your right elbow towards your left knee as you twist your torso to the left.

3. Release and repeat on the opposite side.

Benefits: This exercise targets the obliques and core, building muscle strength and endurance in these areas.

Wall-assisted Reverse Crunch
1. Lie on your back facing a wall, with your hands on the wall at shoulder height, fingers pointing forward.

2. Bring your knees towards your chest, lifting your hips off the ground.

3. Release and repeat for desired number of repetitions.

Benefits: This exercise targets the lower abs, building muscle strength and endurance in this area.

Wall-assisted Scissor Kicks
1. Lie on your back facing a wall, with your hands on the wall at shoulder height, fingers pointing forward.

2. Lift your legs off the ground and kick them back and forth, crossing one over the other.

3. Repeat for desired number of repetitions.

Benefits: This exercise targets the lower abs, building muscle strength and endurance in this area.

CHAPTER 6: ADVANCED WALL PILATES FOR SENIORS

Progressing To More Challenging Exercises

Wall-assisted One-legged Squats

1. Stand with your back against a wall, with your feet hip-width apart and about a foot away from the wall.

2. Shift your weight onto one leg and lift the other leg off the ground, keeping your knee bent.

3. Slowly bend your standing leg, lowering your body towards the ground as if you're sitting back into a chair.

4. Keep your back against the wall and your chest lifted.

5. Push through your heel to straighten your leg and return to the starting position.

6. Repeat for desired reps and then switch legs.

Benefits: This exercise targets the quadriceps, hamstrings, glutes, and core, working on balance, stability and building strength and endurance in the legs.

Wall-assisted One-legged Lunges

1. Stand with your back against a wall, with your feet hip-width apart and about a foot away from the wall.

2. Step forward with one leg, keeping your back against the wall.

3. Bend both knees to lower your body towards the ground, keeping your front knee aligned with your ankle.

4. Push through your front heel to return to the starting position.

5. Repeat for desired reps and then switch legs.

Benefits: This exercise targets the quadriceps, hamstrings, glutes, and core, working on balance, stability and building strength and endurance in the legs and core.

Wall-assisted Handstand Push-ups

1. Start in a handstand position with your hands against a wall and your feet on the ground.

2. Lower your body towards the wall, keeping your elbows close to your body.

3. Push through your hands to return to the starting position.

Benefits: This exercise targets the shoulders, triceps, and core, building upper body strength and increasing shoulder stability.

Wall-assisted Dips with leg raise

1. Place your hands on a wall, shoulder-width apart, and extend your legs out in front of you.
2. Lower your body towards the wall by bending your elbows, keeping them close to your body.

3. Push through your hands to return to the starting position.

4. As you push up, lift one leg off the ground.

5. Repeat for desired reps and then switch legs.

Benefits: This exercise targets the triceps, shoulders, and core, building upper body strength and stability while also working on core and leg strength.

Wall-assisted Plank Jacks

1. Start in a plank position with your hands on a wall and your feet on the ground.

2. Jump your feet out to the sides, keeping your body in a straight line.

3. Jump your feet back to the starting position.

Benefits: This exercise targets the shoulders, triceps, core, and legs, building upper body and core strength and endurance.

Wall-assisted Burpees

1. Start in a standing position with your feet hip-width apart and about a foot away from a wall.

2. Squat down and place your hands on the ground in front of you.

3. Jump your feet back into a plank position, with your hands still on the ground.

4. Jump your feet back up towards your hands.

5. Jump up, reaching your hands towards the ceiling.

6. Repeat.

Benefits: This exercise targets the full-body, working on cardio and building strength and endurance in the legs, core, and upper body.

Wall-assisted Spiderman Push-ups

1. Start in a plank position with your hands on a wall and your feet on the ground.

2. Lower your body towards the wall by bending your elbows, keeping them close to your body.

3. As you push up, bring one knee towards the opposite elbow.

4. Return to the starting position and repeat on the other side.

Benefits: This exercise targets the chest, shoulders, triceps, and core, building upper body strength and stability while also working on core and leg strength.

Wall-assisted Tuck Jumps

1. Stand facing a wall with your feet hip-width apart and about a foot away from the wall.

2. Lower into a squat position, then jump up, bringing your knees towards your chest.

3. Land softly and immediately lower back into a squat to prepare for the next jump.

Benefits: This exercise targets the legs and core, building strength and endurance in the legs and core, and working on explosive power.

Wall-assisted Plyometric Push-ups
1. Start in a plank position with your hands on a wall and your feet on the ground.

2. Lower your body towards the wall by bending your elbows, keeping them close to your body.

3. Push through your hands to return to the starting position, but instead of stopping, push up explosively, lifting your hands off the wall.

4. Land softly and immediately lower back into a plank to prepare for the next rep.

Benefits: This exercise targets the chest, shoulders, triceps, and core, building upper body strength and stability while also working on explosive power.

Wall-assisted Jump Squats
1. Stand facing a wall with your feet hip-width apart and about a foot away from the wall.

2. Lower into a squat position, then jump up explosively.

3. Land softly and immediately lower back into a squat to prepare for the next jump.

Benefits: This exercise targets the legs and core, building strength and endurance in the legs and core, and working on explosive power.

Wall-assisted Box Jumps
1. Stand facing a wall with your feet hip-width apart and about a foot away from the wall.

2. Jump up onto the wall, landing with both feet on the wall.

3. Step down and repeat.

Benefits: This exercise targets the legs and core, building strength and endurance in the legs and core, and working on explosive power.

Wall-assisted Pull-ups with leg raise
1. Hang from a wall with your hands shoulder-width apart.

2. Pull your body up towards the wall, keeping your elbows close to your body.

3. As you pull up, lift one leg off the ground.

4. Lower your body back down, repeat for desired reps and then switch legs.

Benefits: This exercise targets the back, shoulders, and core, building upper body strength and stability while also working on core and leg strength.

Wall-assisted Shoulder press with leg raise
1. Stand facing a wall with your feet hip-width apart and about a foot away from the wall.

2. Place your hands on the wall, shoulder-width apart.

3. Push up, lifting your body off the ground, keeping your back against the wall.

4. As you push up, lift one leg off the ground.

5. Lower your body back down, repeat for desired reps and then switch legs.

Benefits: This exercise targets the shoulders, triceps, and core, building upper body strength and stability while also working on core and leg strength.

Wall-assisted Tricep Dips with leg raise

1. Place your hands on a wall, shoulder-width apart, and extend your legs out in front of you.

2. Lower your body towards the wall by bending your elbows, keeping them close to your body.

3. Push through your hands to return to the starting position.

4. As you push up, lift one leg off the ground.

5. Repeat for desired reps and then switch legs.

Benefits: This exercise targets the triceps, shoulders, and core, building upper body strength and stability while also working on core and leg strength.

Wall-assisted Chest Fly with leg raise
1. Stand facing a wall with your feet hip-width apart and about a foot away from the wall.

2. Place your hands on the wall, shoulder-width apart.

3. Push outwards, lifting your body off the ground, keeping your back against the wall.

4. As you push outwards, lift one leg off the ground.
5. Bring your body back to the center and repeat for desired reps and then switch legs.

Benefits: This exercise targets the chest, shoulders, and core, building upper body strength and stability while also working on core and leg strength.

Wall-assisted Lateral raises with leg raise
1. Stand facing a wall with your feet hip-width apart and about a foot away from the wall.

2. Place your hands on the wall, shoulder-width apart.

3. Push outwards, lifting your body off the ground, keeping your back against the wall.

4. As you push outwards, lift one leg off the ground and raise it to the side.

5. Bring your body back to the center and repeat for desired reps and then switch legs.

Benefits: This exercise targets the shoulders, and core, building upper body strength and stability while also working on core and leg strength.

Wall-assisted Reverse Fly with leg raise

1. Stand facing a wall with your feet hip-width apart and about a foot away from the wall.

2. Place your hands on the wall, shoulder-width apart, and extend your arms out to the sides.

3. Push outwards, lifting your body off the ground, keeping your back against the wall.

4. As you push outwards, lift one leg off the ground and raise it behind you.

5. Bring your body back to the center and repeat for desired reps and then switch legs.

Benefits: This exercise targets the shoulders, and core, building upper body strength and stability while also working on core and leg strength.

Wall-assisted Russian Twist with leg raise
1. Sit facing a wall with your feet hip-width apart and about a foot away from the wall.

2. Place your hands on the wall, shoulder-width apart.

3. Twist your torso to the right, keeping your hands on the wall.

4. As you twist, lift one leg off the ground and raise it to the opposite side of your torso.

5. Twist to the left and repeat for desired reps and then switch legs.

Benefits: This exercise targets the oblique, and core, building core strength and stability while also working on core and leg strength.

Wall-assisted Crunch with leg raise

1. Sit facing a wall with your feet hip-width apart and about a foot away from the wall.

2. Place your hands on the wall, shoulder-width apart.

3. Crunch your torso forward, keeping your hands on the wall.

4. As you crunch, lift one leg off the ground and raise it to the opposite side of your torso.

5. Repeat for desired reps and then switch legs.

Benefits: This exercise targets the abdominal muscles, and core, building core strength and stability while also working on core and leg strength.

Wall-assisted Leg Raise with leg raise
1. Lie facing a wall with your feet hip-width apart and about a foot away from the wall.

2. Place your hands on the wall, shoulder-width apart.

3. Raise both legs off the ground, keeping your hands on the wall.
4. As you raise, lift one leg off the ground and raise it to the opposite side of your torso.

5. Lower your legs and repeat for desired reps and then switch legs.

Benefits: This exercise targets the abdominal muscles and core, building core strength and stability while also working on core and leg strength.

Note: These exercises are considered as advanced exercises, it's important to build up to them gradually.

Incorporating Props For Added Resistance

Wall-assisted Push-ups with resistance bands

Stand facing the wall and place the resistance band around your back, at the level of your chest. Hold the band with your hands and step back to create tension in the band. Start in a plank position, with your hands on the wall, and your feet on the floor. Keep your body straight and your core engaged. Lower your chest towards the wall by bending your elbows, then press back up to the starting position. Repeat the movement for the desired number of reps. This exercise will help to target your chest, triceps and shoulders, and improve your upper body strength.

Wall-assisted Squats with resistance bands

Stand facing the wall with your feet shoulder-width apart. Place the resistance band around your thighs, just above your knees. Hold the band with your hands and step back to create tension in the band. Start with your feet shoulder-width apart and your toes pointing forward. Keep your back straight and your core engaged. Lower your body by bending your knees, then press back up to the starting position. Repeat the movement for the desired number of reps. This exercise will help to target your quadriceps, glutes, and hamstrings, and improve your lower body strength.

Wall-assisted Lunges with resistance bands

Stand facing the wall with your feet shoulder-width apart. Place the resistance band around your thighs, just above your knees. Hold the band with your hands and step back to create tension in the band. Step forward with your right foot, lowering your body by bending your right knee. Keep your back straight and your core engaged. Push back to the starting position, then repeat the movement with your left leg. Repeat the movement for the desired number of reps. This exercise will help to target your quadriceps, glutes, and hamstrings, and improve your lower body strength and balance.

Wall-assisted Tricep Dips with weights

Stand facing the wall and place your hands on the wall, shoulder-width apart. Hold a weight in each hand and lower your body by bending your elbows. Keep your back straight and your core engaged. Push back to the starting position, then repeat the movement for the desired number of reps. This exercise will help to target your triceps and improve your upper body strength.

Wall-assisted Leg Raises with weights

Stand facing the wall and place your hands on the wall, shoulder-width apart. Hold a weight in each hand and raise your right leg off the floor. Keep your back straight and your core engaged. Lower your right leg back down to the starting position, then repeat the movement with your left leg. Repeat the movement for the desired number of reps. This exercise will help to target your lower abs and improve your core strength.

Wall-assisted Shoulder press with dumbbells

Stand facing the wall and place your hands on the wall, shoulder-width apart. Hold a dumbbell in each hand and press the weights up over your head. Keep your back straight and your core engaged. Lower the weights back down to the starting position, then repeat the movement for the desired number of reps. This exercise will help to target your shoulders and improve your upper body strength.

Wall-assisted Bicep Curls with dumbbells

Stand facing the wall and place your hands on the wall, shoulder-width apart. Hold a dumbbell in each hand and curl the weights up towards your shoulders. Keep your back straight and your core engaged. Lower the weights back down to the starting position, then repeat the movement for the desired number of reps. This exercise will help to target your bicep and improve your upper body strength.

Wall-assisted Chest Fly with dumbbells

Stand facing the wall and place your hands on the wall, shoulder-width apart. Hold a dumbbell in each hand and press the weights up over your head. Keep your back straight and your core engaged. Lower the weights out to the sides, keeping your elbows slightly bent. Bring the weights back to the starting position, then repeat the movement for the desired number of reps. This exercise will help to target your chest and improve your upper body strength.

Wall-assisted Lateral raises with dumbbells

Stand facing the wall and place your hands on the wall, shoulder-width apart. Hold a dumbbell in each hand and raise the weights out to the sides, keeping your elbows slightly bent. Keep your back straight and your core engaged. Lower the weights back down to the starting position, then repeat the movement for the desired number of reps. This exercise will help to target your shoulders and improve your upper body strength.

Wall-assisted Upright Rows with dumbbells

Stand facing the wall and place your hands on the wall, shoulder-width apart. Hold a dumbbell in each hand and raise the weights up towards your shoulders, keeping your elbows pointed out to the sides. Keep your back straight and your core engaged. Lower the weights back down to the starting position, then repeat the movement for the desired number of reps. This exercise will help to target your shoulders and improve your upper body strength.

Wall-assisted Lat Pull-downs with resistance bands

Stand facing the wall and place the resistance band above your head, with the band anchored to the wall. Hold the band with your hands and step back to create tension in the band. Keep your back straight and your core engaged. Pull the band down towards your chest, then release back to the starting position. Repeat the movement for the desired number of reps. This exercise will help to target your back and improve your upper body strength.

Wall-assisted Seated Row with resistance bands

Stand facing the wall and place the resistance band around your back, at the level of your chest. Hold the band with your hands and step back to create tension in the band. Keep your back straight and your core engaged. Pull the band towards your chest, then release back to the starting position. Repeat the movement for the desired number of reps. This exercise will help to target your back and improve your upper body strength.

Wall-assisted Reverse Fly with dumbbells

Stand facing the wall and place your hands on the wall, shoulder-width apart. Hold a dumbbell in each hand and press the weights up over your head. Keep your back straight and your core engaged. Lower the weights out to the sides, keeping your elbows slightly bent. Bring the weights back to the starting position, then repeat the movement for the desired number of reps. This exercise will help to target your shoulders and improve your upper body strength.

Wall-assisted Plank hold with resistance bands

Stand facing the wall and place the resistance band around your back, at the level of your chest. Hold the band with your hands and step back to create tension in the band. Start in a plank position, with your hands on the wall, and your feet on the floor. Keep your body straight and your core engaged. Hold the position for the desired amount of time, then release. Repeat the movement for the desired number of reps. This exercise will help to target your core and improve your overall body strength.

Wall-assisted Side Plank with weights

Stand facing the wall and place your left hand on the wall, shoulder-width apart. Hold a weight in your right hand and raise your hips off the floor, balancing on your left hand and your left foot. Keep your body straight and your core engaged. Hold the position for the desired amount of time, then release. Repeat the movement for the desired number of reps on each side. This exercise will help to target your obliques and improve your overall body strength and balance.

Wall-assisted Russian Twist with weights

Stand facing the wall and place your hands on the wall, shoulder-width apart. Hold a weight in your right hand and twist your torso to the left, keeping your back straight and your core engaged. Return to the starting position, then repeat the movement on the opposite side. Repeat the movement for the desired number of reps. This exercise will help to target your obliques and improve your overall body strength and balance.

Wall-assisted Crunch with resistance bands

Stand facing the wall and place the resistance band around your back, at the level of your chest. Hold the band with your hands and step back to create tension in the band. Lie down on the floor and place your feet on the wall, keeping your back straight and your core engaged. Crunch your torso up towards the wall, then release back to the starting position. Repeat the movement for the desired number of reps. This exercise will help to target your abs and improve your overall body strength.

Wall-assisted Leg Raise with resistance bands

Stand facing the wall and place the resistance band around your back, at the level of your chest. Hold the band with your hands and step back to create tension in the band. Lie down on the floor and place your feet on the wall, keeping your back straight and your core engaged. Raise your legs up towards the wall, then release back to the starting position. Repeat the movement for the desired number of reps. This exercise will help to target your lower abs and improve your overall body strength.

Wall-assisted Bicycle Crunch with resistance bands

Stand facing the wall and place the resistance band around your back, at the level of your chest. Hold the band with your hands and step back to create tension in the band. Lie down on the floor and place your feet on the wall, keeping your back straight and your core engaged. Crunch your torso up towards the wall, and twist your torso to the left, bringing your right elbow towards your left knee. Alternate sides, then release back to the starting position. Repeat the movement for the desired number of reps. This exercise will help to target your abs and improve your overall body strength and balance.

Wall-assisted Reverse Crunch with resistance bands

Stand facing the wall and place the resistance band around your back, at the level of your chest. Hold the band with your hands and step back to create tension in the band. Lie down on the floor and place your feet on the wall, keeping your back straight and your core engaged. Crunch your hips up towards the wall, then release back to the starting position. Repeat the movement for the desired number of reps. This exercise will help to target your lower abs and improve your overall body strength.

CHAPTER 7: INCORPORATING WALL PILATES INTO YOUR DAILY ROUTINE

Tips For Making Wall Pilates A Part Of Your Daily Routine

Start with a clear goal in mind: Decide what you want to achieve from your Wall Pilates routine and set a clear goal to work towards.

Create a schedule: Set aside a specific time of day for your Wall Pilates routine and make it a part of your daily schedule.

Start small: Start with a few basic exercises and gradually increase the intensity and duration of your routine as you build strength and endurance.

Mix it up: Don't stick to the same routine every day. Mix things up by incorporating different exercises and props to keep your routine interesting and challenging.

Listen to your body: Be mindful of your body's limitations and don't push yourself too hard. If you feel pain or discomfort, take a break or stop the exercise.

Track your progress: Keep a log of your progress and celebrate your achievements along the way.

Incorporate other forms of exercise: Wall Pilates is a great way to improve flexibility, balance, and strength, but it's essential to incorporate other forms of exercise, such as cardio, to maintain overall fitness and health.

Have fun: Remember to enjoy the process and have fun! Wall Pilates is a fantastic way to improve your overall wellness, and it's essential to enjoy the journey.

Make it a part of your daily routine: Incorporate Wall Pilates into your daily routine, this way you'll be more likely to stick to it in the long run.

Set realistic expectations: It's important to set realistic expectations for yourself and understand that progress takes time. Be patient with yourself and trust the process.

Be consistent: Consistency is key when it comes to making Wall Pilates a part of your daily routine. Try to stick to your schedule as much as possible and don't give up too easily.

Find a workout partner: Having a workout partner can help to motivate and encourage you to stick to your routine. Find a friend or family member who is interested in Wall Pilates and work out together.

Stay hydrated and well-nourished: Proper hydration and nutrition are essential for optimal performance and recovery. Make sure you are drinking enough water and eating a healthy diet to fuel your workouts.

Take rest days: It's important to give your body time to recover and rest. Make sure you take at least one rest day a week to allow your muscles to recover and prevent injury.

Reward yourself: Set up a reward system for yourself to keep you motivated. For example, after completing a certain number of workouts, treat yourself to a massage or a new piece of workout gear.

Take it slow: Remember to take it slow and don't push yourself too hard. If you're new to Wall Pilates, start with short, easy exercises and gradually increase the intensity as you build strength and endurance.

Be open-minded: Be open-minded to new exercises and variations. Wall Pilates offers a wide range of exercises that can be tailored to your needs and preferences.

Keep a positive mindset: Stay positive and believe in yourself. With time, patience and practice, you'll see the benefits of Wall Pilates for seniors and make it a permanent part of your daily routine.

Sample Workout Plans

Sample Workout Plan 1: Beginner's Wall Pilates Routine

Monday:

Wall-assisted hamstring stretch: Hold for 30 seconds, rest for 15 seconds, repeat 3 times

Wall-assisted hip flexor stretch: Hold for 30 seconds, rest for 15 seconds, repeat 3 times

Wall-assisted quad stretch: Hold for 30 seconds, rest for 15 seconds, repeat 3 times

Wall-assisted inner thigh stretch: Hold for 30 seconds, rest for 15 seconds, repeat 3 times

Wall-assisted calf stretch: Hold for 30 seconds, rest for 15 seconds, repeat 3 times

Wall-assisted ankle stretch: Hold for 30 seconds, rest for 15 seconds, repeat 3 times

Tuesday:

Wall-assisted standing hamstring stretch: Hold for 30 seconds, rest for 15 seconds, repeat 3 times

Wall-assisted standing hip flexor stretch: Hold for 30 seconds, rest for 15 seconds, repeat 3 times

Wall-assisted standing quad stretch: Hold for 30 seconds, rest for 15 seconds, repeat 3 times

Wall-assisted standing inner thigh stretch: Hold for 30 seconds, rest for 15 seconds, repeat 3 times

Wall-assisted standing calf stretch: Hold for 30 seconds, rest for 15 seconds, repeat 3 times

Wall-assisted standing ankle stretch: Hold for 30 seconds, rest for 15 seconds, repeat 3 times

Wednesday: Rest Day

Thursday:

Wall-assisted hamstring stretch: Hold for 30 seconds, rest for 15 seconds, repeat 3 times

Wall-assisted hip flexor stretch: Hold for 30 seconds, rest for 15 seconds, repeat 3 times

Wall-assisted quad stretch: Hold for 30 seconds, rest for 15 seconds, repeat 3 times

Wall-assisted inner thigh stretch: Hold for 30 seconds, rest for 15 seconds, repeat 3 times

Wall-assisted calf stretch: Hold for 30 seconds, rest for 15 seconds, repeat 3 times

Wall-assisted ankle stretch: Hold for 30 seconds, rest for 15 seconds, repeat 3 times

Friday:

Wall-assisted standing hamstring stretch: Hold for 30 seconds, rest for 15 seconds, repeat 3 times

Wall-assisted standing hip flexor stretch: Hold for 30 seconds, rest for 15 seconds, repeat 3 times

Wall-assisted standing quad stretch: Hold for 30 seconds, rest for 15 seconds, repeat 3 times

Wall-assisted standing inner thigh stretch: Hold for 30 seconds, rest for 15 seconds, repeat 3 times

Wall-assisted standing calf stretch: Hold for 30 seconds, rest for 15 seconds, repeat 3 times

Wall-assisted standing ankle stretch: Hold for 30 seconds, rest for 15 seconds, repeat 3 times

Saturday: Rest Day

Sunday:

Wall-assisted hamstring stretch: Hold for 30 seconds, rest for 15 seconds, repeat 3 times

Wall-assisted hip flexor stretch: Hold for 30 seconds, rest for 15 seconds, repeat 3 times

Wall-assisted quad stretch: Hold for 30 seconds, rest for 15 seconds, repeat 3 times

Wall-assisted inner thigh stretch: Hold for 30 seconds, rest for 15 seconds, repeat 3 times

Wall-assisted calf stretch: Hold for 30 seconds, rest for 15 seconds, repeat 3 times

Wall-assisted ankle stretch: Hold for 30 seconds, rest for 15 seconds, repeat 3 times

This routine should be done 3 days a week, with at least one rest day in between each workout.

Sample Workout Plan 2: Intermediate Wall Pilates Routine

Monday:

Wall-assisted push-ups: 3 sets of 10 reps, rest for 30 seconds between sets

Wall-assisted squats: 3 sets of 10 reps, rest for 30 seconds between sets

Wall-assisted lunges: 3 sets of 10 reps, rest for 30 seconds between sets

Wall-assisted tricep dips: 3 sets of 10 reps, rest for 30 seconds between sets

Wall-assisted leg raises: 3 sets of 10 reps, rest for 30 seconds between sets

Wall-assisted squat holds: 3 sets of 30 seconds, rest for 15 seconds between sets

Wall-assisted hamstring curls: 3 sets of 10 reps, rest for 30 seconds between sets

Wall-assisted calf raises: 3 sets of 10 reps, rest for 30 seconds between sets

Wall-assisted side planks: 3 sets of 30 seconds, rest for 15 seconds between sets

Wall-assisted shoulder taps: 3 sets of 10 reps, rest for 30 seconds between sets

Tuesday:

Wall-assisted Pull-ups: 3 sets of 10 reps, rest for 30 seconds between sets

Wall-assisted Rows: 3 sets of 10 reps, rest for 30 seconds between sets

Wall-assisted Shoulder Press: 3 sets of 10 reps, rest for 30 seconds between sets

Wall-assisted Bicep Curls: 3sets of 10 reps, rest for 30 seconds between sets

Wall-assisted Tricep Dips: 3 sets of 10 reps, rest for 30 seconds between sets

Wall-assisted Chest Fly: 3 sets of 10 reps, rest for 30 seconds between sets

Wall-assisted Chest Press: 3 sets of 10 reps, rest for 30 seconds between sets

Wall-assisted Lateral Raises: 3 sets of 10 reps, rest for 30 seconds between sets

Wall-assisted Upright Rows: 3 sets of 10 reps, rest for 30 seconds between sets

Wall-assisted Lat Pull-downs: 3 sets of 10 reps, rest for 30 seconds between sets

Wednesday: Rest Day

Thursday:

Wall-assisted push-ups: 3 sets of 10 reps, rest for 30 seconds between sets

Wall-assisted squats: 3 sets of 10 reps, rest for 30 seconds between sets

Wall-assisted lunges: 3 sets of 10 reps, rest for 30 seconds between sets

Wall-assisted tricep dips: 3 sets of 10 reps, rest for 30 seconds between sets

Wall-assisted leg raises: 3 sets of 10 reps, rest for 30 seconds between sets

Wall-assisted squat holds: 3 sets of 30 seconds, rest for 15 seconds between sets

Wall-assisted hamstring curls: 3 sets of 10 reps, rest for 30 seconds between sets

Wall-assisted calf raises: 3 sets of 10 reps, rest for 30 seconds between sets

Wall-assisted side planks: 3 sets of 30 seconds, rest for 15 seconds between sets

Wall-assisted shoulder taps: 3 sets of 10 reps, rest for 30 seconds between sets

Friday:

Wall-assisted Pull-ups: 3 sets of 10 reps, rest for 30 seconds between sets

Wall-assisted Rows: 3 sets of10 reps, rest for 30 seconds between sets

Wall-assisted Shoulder Press: 3 sets of 10 reps, rest for 30 seconds between sets

Wall-assisted Bicep Curls: 3 sets of 10 reps, rest for 30 seconds between sets

Wall-assisted Tricep Dips: 3 sets of 10 reps, rest for 30 seconds between sets

Wall-assisted Chest Fly: 3 sets of 10 reps, rest for 30 seconds between sets

Wall-assisted Chest Press: 3 sets of 10 reps, rest for 30 seconds between sets

Wall-assisted Lateral Raises: 3 sets of 10 reps, rest for 30 seconds between sets

Wall-assisted Upright Rows: 3 sets of 10 reps, rest for 30 seconds between sets

Wall-assisted Lat Pull-downs: 3 sets of 10 reps, rest for 30 seconds between sets

Saturday: Rest Day

Sunday:

Wall-assisted push-ups: 3 sets of 10 reps, rest for 30 seconds between sets

Wall-assisted squats: 3 sets of 10 reps, rest for 30 seconds between sets

Wall-assisted lunges: 3 sets of 10 reps, rest for 30 seconds between sets

Wall-assisted tricep dips: 3 sets of 10 reps, rest for 30 seconds between sets

Wall-assisted leg raises: 3 sets of 10 reps, rest for 30 seconds between sets

Wall-assisted squat holds: 3 sets of 30 seconds, rest for 15 seconds between sets

Wall-assisted hamstring curls: 3 sets of 10 reps, rest for 30 seconds between sets

Wall-assisted calf raises: 3 sets of 10 reps, rest for 30 seconds between sets

Wall-assisted side planks: 3 sets of 30 seconds, rest for 15 seconds between sets

Wall-assisted shoulder taps: 3 sets of 10 reps, rest for 30 seconds between sets

This routine should be done 3 days a week, with at least one rest day in between each workout.

It's important to note that the duration of each exercise, rest time between each set and how many days a week the routine should be done, can be adjusted to suit the needs and abilities of the individual.

Printed in Great Britain
by Amazon

20943990R10088